The Keto Slow Cooker Cookbook

Quick and easy Ketogenic Diet Recipes for Rapid Weight Loss & Burn Fat Forever (Crock Pot Cookbook for Beginners and Pros)

Jason Cooker

Table of Contents

Introduction

Deciding to go on the ketogenic diet is an easy decision for some and more challenging for others. Chances are if you've bought this cookbook, you've already decided, then congratulations! Dieting is never the easiest road, but these recipes make it easier by giving you back some of that deliciousness you may have missed out on with other diets. Not only that, but these recipes are an introduction to a whole new lifestyle of healthiness.

Going on a keto diet means you have to cook most of your meals at home, as most foods served in eating places are not keto-friendly. Many of us have a day-job, so cooking may become a chore. After you come home exhausted from a workday, the thought of cooking is not a pleasant one. So, the slow cooker comes to the rescue, to those who want and wishes to eat nutritious Keto meals can now come home with food ready to eat. While you are working at the office or doing other chores, cooking your food will be unattended in your kitchen with the magic of your slow cooker.

The fantastic slow cooker allows you to prepare the ingredients in the morning and have it ready for lunch or dinner. Or you can even let it cook while you sleep so you can wake up to an excellent ready breakfast. You can even pack some of it for your lunch at work.

For example, you can cook your favorite pulled pork overnight to supply the meat needed for a keto-friendly wrap using lettuce or omelette and pack it as your lunch after you had your breakfast. Or you can make meatballs during the day and save some for breakfast (freeze in your fridge after cooking) for the next morning.

For it to make even more time saving, many ingredients can be prepared the night before. Chopped the necessary ingredients, put them in airtight containers or Ziplock bags, and store in the fridge overnight to speed things along in the morning. In the morning, before you leave work, pour the ingredients into the pot out and turn on your slow cooker and start cooking. Hence, the slow cooker is an indispensable cooking gadget for those doing the keto diet.

Other benefits that the slow cooker will provide you are:

- Save Electricity: Compared to the oven, the slow-cooker uses less electricity. On low, it runs on the same amount of energy needed to power a 75 to a 100-watt light bulb.
- Lower heat production: Your house is not going to get warm, unlike using an oven, and you don't have to fear that your house will burn down due to overheating. The slow-cooker is safe to leave to its own devices without any supervision, unlike dishes left in the oven or on the stovetop.
- More meat choices: You can now include tougher meat on your menu. The slow, moist cooking environment breaks the tough tissue of less tender, but very affordable, cuts of meat—the portions of muscle used the most, such as the chuck, brisket, round, and shank. It is perfect for cooking lamb shanks!
- High nutritious food: The slow-cooking of bones and meats melt collagens that enrich the dish's liquid with its flavor and many nutrients. It is perfect for making healthy and delicious soups.
- In this cookbook, we will go in-depth first with Keto history and how it works, then we will get to know your slow cooker and how to use it, and finally, we will provide you 200 Keto-friendly recipes that will surely bring your slow cooker at its best.

Using a slow-cooker is just one of the added benefits of these recipes. They'll be more tender, more flavorful, and much easier to prepare than ordinary stovetop or oven meals. They'll allow you to spend less time in the kitchen and more quality time with your family. So, get ready for some serious yumminess in your life and a Keto diet that no one will object to!

CHAPTER 1:

The Keto History & How Does It Work

It might shock and surprise you to know that the keto diet was in popular use as early as the 1920s and 1930s. At least, this is when it became popular as an alternative treatment for those who had epilepsy.

The keto diet was introduced as a therapy for those with epilepsy, as studies had shown that recent fasting methods had helped reduce the severity of the condition. As other anticonvulsant therapies (such as new medications) became available, the keto diet was almost all but forgotten about.

Unfortunately, when the medications were unable to help around 30 percent of those with epilepsy, the ketogenic diet was re-introduced. It is still used as a recommendation today for those with epilepsy—particularly children—as its effects have always proven to help reduce and manage the seizures caused by epilepsy.

There were many years where doctors discovered more about the benefits of entering a ketosis state for epilepsy. The treatment for epilepsy with fasting or a low carb diet dates back to ancient Greek physicians' times. In 1921, an endocrinologist named Rollin Woodyat found the three water-soluble compounds in the liver known today as ketones. Dr. Rollin Woodyat noted that the liver was producing the ketone molecules as a result of fasting.

The same year that Woodyat found where the ketone molecules were being made, the diet received its official name from Russel Wilder and the Mayo Clinic before it was commonly used as an epileptic treatment. Shortly after anticonvulsant drugs became popular, doctors no longer received training in the keto diet. It caused a few doctors that tried to use it to implement it incorrectly. For optimal results with the keto diet, it is crucial to use it appropriately and follow it as needed to trigger ketone molecules' production and release.

While the ketogenic diet took off in popularity as a therapy for epilepsy patients, it did not pass by unnoticed the effect it had on weight loss. Even though the keto diet almost disappeared due to a lack of use, around the 1990s, it made a reappearance. It began to grow more in notoriety for weight loss in the early 2000s.

After the 2000s, the keto diet took off in popularity and since then has been successfully used by thousands for weight loss. In recent years the keto diet has taken off due to its advantages in the health field. The benefits of the keto diet are linked to sustained weight loss and epilepsy, and other medical issues are reported to improve with the use of this diet.

How Does Ketosis Work

Now you know how the ketogenic diet came into popularity and that it is achieved by entering into a metabolic state known as ketosis. But how exactly does this work?

When you enter the state of ketosis, you are cutting your body off of its glucose supply. It means that to complete those vital life functions like breathing, your body needs to find a different fuel source.

When you fast or drastically reduce the number of carbs you eat, you limit your body's glucose. Low levels of glucose send an indicator to the body that it needs to produce energy.

It triggers the body to enter the metabolic state of ketosis. This state can take anywhere from three days to one week to obtain. There is some indication you might be feeling during this period, which we will go over later in this guide. Once you are in the ketosis state, your liver transforms your fat cells into ketone molecules. These ketone molecules are a supplement energy cell to glucose.

Since the keto diet relies on your fat for energy, this is where sustained weight loss comes into play. Because your body and brain will now depend on fat processed through the liver into ketones for energy, it will begin to break down and use the stored fat on your body in the same way. How amazing is that?

Once your body has entered its full metabolic state of ketosis, the result will be a lowered production of glucose and an increase in fat breakdown. There will be some specific signals that indicate your body has entered ketosis, which we will go over next.

So, how do you know when your body has entered ketosis? It can take anywhere from 3 days to a week (depending on how you ease yourself into the keto diet) to achieve the state of ketosis. There are signs or symptoms to help you understand what is going on with your body and where you change from using glucose to ketone molecules for fuel.

One of the symptoms that your body is in the full state of ketosis is bad breath. Most people report that their breath takes on a fruity smell or a bad smell when they start the keto diet. It is a good mark because it indicates that you have reached the state of ketosis.

Most people on the keto diet experience bad breath because of the compound acetone, which is found in ketone molecules. The acetone is expelled from the body through urine and breath. So, this is why many reports that they experience bad breath while on the keto diet.

Most people on the keto diet compensate for this by brushing their teeth several times a day and using sugar-free gums or mints. Keep in mind to always check the labels of your gum packets for carbs! You do not want to take your body out of ketosis since you worked hard to get there.

The other sign—probably the one you will be most excited about—is the weight loss from the keto diet. So, unlike other diets where you lose a lot of weight short-term and struggle with long-term goals, the keto will continue to provide weight loss benefits. This initial weight loss is simply the usage of stored carbs and loss of water weight. After this, your weight loss should be consistent over time, as long as you follow the basic outline of your Keto diet. An effective diet follows the program; otherwise, you will not experience the results you want.

Another marker that you are in ketosis is, of course, an increase in blood ketone levels. There are some are tests that you can buy to test your blood ketone levels! They are the easiest way to test your levels for this sign. This test works by testing for a compound called beta-hydroxybutyrate (BHB) in your blood. The test is a meter that looks for the amount of BHB in levels in your blood. BHB is the primary ketone present in the blood. Remember that a ketone consists of three compounds.

The drawback of testing ketones this way is that you have to prick your finger with blood, and the tests can be expensive. But there are other signs to know if your body is in ketosis!

Remember that bad breath we spoke about earlier? Well, let us get back to it. We are sure you have heard of a breathalyzer to test for alcohol limits. We bet you did not know that you can also use the breath analyzer to measure acetone levels in your breath! And since acetone is one of the three main components of ketone molecules, you will find a good sign about your ketosis state with this method.

The way to find out is by monitoring how much acetone exits your body. During the state of ketosis, your body will expel more acetone levels. While this method is less accurate than the blood meter tests mentioned above, it is still a fairly accurate way to determine if you are in nutritional ketosis.

Nutritional ketosis is just the label for your body's metabolic state of ketosis, where fat is burned instead of sugar. You can also get urine strips to measure acetone levels, leaving your body through your urine. These test strips are a cheaper way to test for acetone levels; however, they are not considered to be very reliable.

The reason you might feel sick or sluggish at first is because of the major changes your body is making. You are switching from using sugar as energy to use fat as energy! It requires your body to undergo some changes, and as a result, you might not feel your best in the first week of the keto diet.

But the long-term results and studies all point to significant increases in both focus and energy when following the keto diet. The reason for this is because ketone molecules are a powerful fuel source for the brain. They have even been used in studies regarding concussions and memory loss.

As mentioned above, some people experience tiredness when they start the keto diet. This symptom is only for the short-term, and it, too, is a good sign that you are in the beginning stages of nutritional ketosis.

This symptom is often the hardest for people to manage, and one of the main reasons they tend to quit the keto diet before realizing its true benefits and rewards. Keep in mind that this is normal to experience. Your body has been used to running on carbohydrates, and the switch to ketones can be taxing on your body.

Because the keto diet involves major changes to the ordinary diet, expect a few digestive issues to follow. Constipation and diarrhea are common during this stage, as they are common symptoms that follow any major dietary shift. Once the transitional changes are over, these symptoms should stop.

To ensure that your body's systems remain running as smoothly as possible, be mindful to eat vegetables that contain a lot of fiber.

The final most common symptom that comes from the initial diet change is insomnia. Many people experience insomnia or wake up in the middle of the night, having difficulty getting back to sleep at night when they switch their diet to the keto diet. It is mainly due to the drastic reduction in carbohydrates.

Once you are adapted to your new keto diet, your sleep should improve in the long-term. With the keto diet, you must note it is not about short-term goals. While there are many health benefits to the keto diet, this can be a lifestyle change! So, the benefits you are looking for are on a long-term plan. But these benefits are achievable and within reach of anyone who follows the ketogenic diet.

CHAPTER 2:

The Slow Cooker

Regardless of your initial opinion of diets, in general, it is essential to promote the view that the primary purpose of the keto diet is your ultimate health and the health of your family and loved ones. When people think of cooking ingredients, even when they are whole foods, they usually stick to the most traditional boiling, frying, or roasting methods. The problem with these ways of cooking food is that most people will overdo it, and as a result, will destroy all of the healthy nutrients of the whole foods that they spent their hard-earned money purchasing. Sometimes, the cook doesn't have enough experience in the kitchen, and sometimes it's just because there is a lack of patience after a long workday. The slow cooker solves all of these problems because it controls the cook without the possibility of an outside source ruining the ingredients inside.

A Quick Note on Recipe Adaptation: Because it has its cooking system, the slow cooker has particular recipes based on it alone. You cannot just take any recipe you find and make it in the slow cooker; however, you can adapt them to suit this appliance. This cookbook will provide you with all the recipes you need to make the most of your slow cooker, so you don't have to worry about altering anything on your own.

The Slow Cooker Requires Little to No Oil

It is one of the healthiest reasons to use a slow cooker. For most recipes, no oil is required at all. For recipes that emulate a 'frying effect,' only a tiny amount of oil is needed to complete the cook. It is important because healthy oils such as olive oil, for example, do not stand high temperatures. Heating it would make it unhealthy. Instead, a tiny amount of coconut oil will do the trick every time. Do not confuse oil with the importance of fat in the keto diet. Although fat is essential, it comes from healthy fat sources such as animal fat or nuts and seeds.

The healthy fat, which is part of the keto diet, does not include cooking oils since their only purpose should be to stop the food from burning.

Your Food Cannot Burn

Provided that you've made all the right settings for the recipe that you are making, the food inside of your slow cooker will never burn. Not only is this because the temperatures inside this appliance will never reach incredibly high levels, but also because its settings will automatically turn the appliance off once the cooking time is up. It is essential for ensuring that your meals never contain carcinogens, which are incredibly unhealthy for anyone.

Self-Made Gravy as an Additional Flavoring

A roast is one of the most popular meals to make in a slow cooker. But traditional gravy, which is almost an essential element to anyone's idea of a Sunday roast, uses flour as a thickening agent. Luckily, this is not the case with a slow cooker. Remember that extra drawer at the bottom of the appliance that collects excess liquid and fat? Those juices can be used as gravy that will go over the top of a roast. It doesn't require any additional ingredients to be thickened, and it is made from the natural juices of the ingredients that you have placed inside the slow cooker, making it a healthy addition to your keto meal.

Easily Cook Beans and Legumes

Beans and legumes are an essential source of protein and healthy fats. However, the problem with these ingredients is that they often take a very long time to prepare because their texture is so hard. Luckily, the slow cooker has the perfect setting specific for these ingredients, so you never have to worry about undercooking or overcooking them. They will be perfect every time with just a little added water. What's also great about the slow cooker combined with these ingredients is that you can pause the cook halfway and add vegetables of your choice for additional texture and flavor. It's a great way to prepare stews for the whole family or a delicious chili recipe.

A Perfect Appliance for All Seasonal Ingredients

Whenever we buy something new in the house, we want to make sure that we can use a good investment in the long run and not just a fad. The slow cooker can prepare any ingredient of your choice all year round. It is essential not only for the vitamins and minerals that you will continuously be able to include in your meals but also for your overall budget, which can often suffer throughout the year if you have to purchase ingredients out of season at higher prices. Every small helps when you are trying to save money for your future and that of your family, and the slow cooker is a great way to use ingredients that are in season, healthy, and at the most beneficial prices.

CHAPTER 3:

How to Use the Slow Cooker?

If you are a newbie to slow cooking, you don't have to worry about any fancy cooking techniques as the slow cooker will work its magic on your own, and the steps of setting up are so easy, even a small kid can cook with it.

When you buy a slow cooker, most manufacturers feature a low or high setting to choose from cooking your food, besides the on/off button. It may vary slightly from every brand, but this is usually the primary setting of a slow cooker. Read the manufacturer's instructions first to make sure you use it properly.

In general, the low setting applies to foods and ingredients that don't need much time to be cooked properly in the oven. In most cases, the low setting should be between ½ to 3 hours max. These are:

- Fish and seafood

- Sausages

- Boneless and skinless or tender cuts of meat, e.g., tenderloin

- Thinly cut veggies

- Soup Mixes

On the other hand, high setting, which takes 3-8 hours in most cases, is suitable for chunkier and tougher veggie or meat pieces like:

- Beef cuts, e.g., steaks, cubes, briskets, prime rib, oxtails

- Pork Chops

- Whole pork shoulders or pork bellies

- Spare ribs

- Celery Stalks

- Carrots (sliced thickly)

As a rule, the more challenging the cut is, the slower cooking time it will need to get juicier and tender—the softer or smallest it is, the less cooking time it will need after setting this on.

For convenience reasons and in a hurry, you can add all the ingredients that a recipe calls chopped (if using meats or veggies) or peeled and wholesome without any other preparation. However, some tips will help you with the best results regarding flavor, texture, and cooking time.

Here are some:

- Brown your meats and veggie chunks first. It is optional, but this helps retain the flavor of meats and veggies and makes them taste more roast instead of boiled. It may sound time-consuming, but it's not—it only takes a couple of minutes on high heat and a bit of oil to get them to change color.
- Use softer ingredients last or in large, thicker pieces. It will ensure that they don't become too mushy or fall apart after slow-cooking. Some green leafy veggies like spinach, which wilt easily, could also be added last (during the last 30 minutes to an hour).
- Fill ideally 2/3 of your slow cooker, so there is a little extra space for the food to cook freely. Filling it too much with solid and liquid ingredients will make the food steamed instead of simmered.
- Layer things properly. Some recipes are all about layering. In general, veggies (especially root vegetables) should come first, followed by meats and then liquids or spices. Don't raise the lid. You may be tempted to take a sneak peek or check if the food has been cooked properly, but if you do this more than once, you will end up losing valuable heat. Some recipes may require

occasional stirring, but lifting the lid is unnecessary and a mistake for most of the recipes.

- Use dairy in moderation. Some dairy products are fine when used in a slow cooker, while others will disintegrate and become a mess, so you better pay attention to the dairy products you add. Hard and fine cheeses like mozzarella and cheddar are fine when added last, but heavy creams and yogurts should be avoided altogether as they will break and fall apart.

- Use alcohol in moderation. While on a regular stovetop, alcohol will evaporate and add its aromas to the food without suffocating it; in a slow cooker using too much alcohol can make food taste just like that—pure, raw alcohol and cover the flavors and aromas of the rest of the dish. A little red or white wine is fine, but anything more than that should be avoided. Don't use poultry (chicken or duck) with the skin on unless you want to end up with a chewy, rubber-like skin that is also flavorless. If you're going to add the skin, you can brown it first on a frying pan to make it a tad crispier and more flavorful. Don't overcook it. Pay close attention to the recipe cooking times and don't overcook something hoping that it will get more tender and juicy—it will only fall apart and become a mushy mess, especially if you are using fish or thinly cut veggies.

- Add the herbs last. Since herbs have a delicate flavor and aroma, putting them in the slow cooker too soon will dilute their scent to the point where you almost don't recognize it. Herbs, just like dairy, are best placed during the last 30 minutes of cooking.

- Finally, make sure you use some stock or any other liquid to submerge lean meat cuts, or your meat will dry up.

CHAPTER 4:

Breakfast

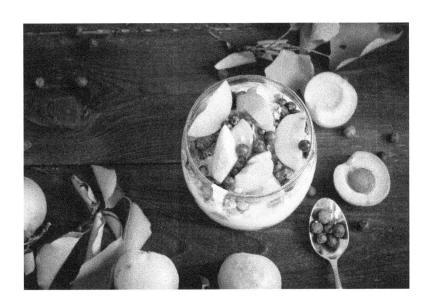

1.   Cauliflower Grits

Preparation time: 5 minutes

Cooking time: 3 hours 15 minutes

Servings: 8

Ingredients:

- 6 cups Cauliflower, chopped into florets

- ½ cup Chicken Stock

- ½ tsp. Black Pepper

- 1 tsp. Sea Salt

- 1 cup Cream Cheese

Directions:

1. Process the cauliflower using a food processor until they are finely processed to 'rice' size. Set it aside. Add all the remaining fixing along with the cauliflower rice into the slow cooker and mix them well. Cook them for 3 hours on low heat. Serve it hot.

Nutrition:

- Calories: 161
- Fat: 10.19g
- Carbohydrates: 3.66g
- Proteins: 3.88g

2.   Broccoli Egg Casserole

time: 10 minutes **Cooking time:** 2 hours 45 minutes **Servings**: 6 to 8

Ingredients:

- 4 cups Broccoli florets, small

- ¼ cup Parmesan Cheese, coarsely grated

- ½ cup Cottage Cheese washed & dried

- 9 Eggs, large & organic

- ½ tsp. Salt

- 6oz. Swiss Cheese

- Black Pepper, as needed, grounded

Directions:

1. First, boil the broccoli florets in a pot of salt water for 2 minutes. Drain well. After that, place the cottage cheese in a strainer and pour cold water above it until the curd remains. Drain well. Then, lightly whisk the egg in another mixing bowl.

2. Now, grease the insides of the slow cooker with butter. Arrange the broccoli florets onto the bottom of the crockpot.

3. Once done, top it with cottage cheese first and then with Swiss cheese. Finally, layer it with the beaten egg and spread it across.

4. Season it with salt and pepper. Garnish it with parmesan cheese and close the lid. Cook on low heat for 2 ½ to 3 hours or until the egg is set.

Nutrition:

- Calories: 220 Fat: 15g Carbohydrates: 3.64g Proteins: 18g

CHAPTER 5:

Lunch

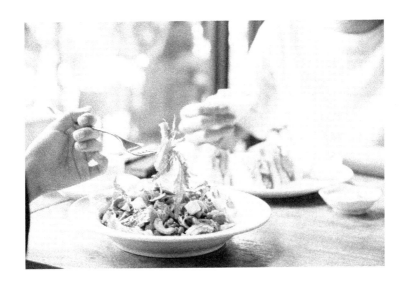

3.   Lemon Thyme Chicken

Preparation time: 15 minutes

Cooking time: 4 hours

Servings: 4

Ingredients:

- 10-15 garlic cloves

- 2 sliced lemons

- ½ teaspoon of ground pepper

- 1 teaspoon of thyme

- 3 ½-pound whole chicken

Directions:

1. Arrange the lemon and garlic on the base of a slow cooker. Mix the spices and use them to season the chicken. Put the chicken in the slow cooker. Cover and cook on low within 4 hours. Remove the chicken, let it stand for 15 minutes, and then serve.

Nutrition:

- Calories: 120
- Fat: 8g
- Carbohydrates: 1g
- Protein: 12g

4. BBQ Ribs

Preparation time: 15 minutes **Cooking time:** 8 hours

Servings: 4

Ingredients:

- 3 pounds of pork ribs

- 1 tablespoon of olive oil

- 1 can of tomato paste, 28 ounces

- ½ cup of hot water

- ½ cup of vinegar

- 6 tablespoons of Worcestershire sauce

- 4 tablespoons of dry mustard

- 1 tablespoon of chili powder

- 1 teaspoon of ground cumin

- 1 teaspoon of powdered sweetener of your choice

- Salt and pepper

Directions:

1. Heat the olive oil in a large frying pan and brown the ribs. Place them in the crockpot. In a small bowl, combine the remaining ingredients, whisk thoroughly and pour over the ribs. Cook for 8 hours on low.

Nutrition: Calories: 410 Carbohydrates: 14g Protein: 38g Fat: 28g

CHAPTER 6:

Dinner

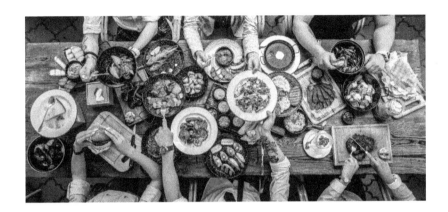

5.   Lemon Garlic Shrimp Scampi

Preparation time: 15 minutes

Cooking time: 1 hour & 30 minutes

Servings: 6

Ingredients:

- 1 lb. raw shrimp, peeled and deveined

- Juice of one fresh lemon

- 1/2 cup chicken broth

- 3 minced garlic cloves

- 4 tbsp butter

- 2 tbsp fresh parsley

- Salt and pepper as desired

Directions:

1. Adjust the heat of the slow cooker to high. Combine the chicken broth, lemon juice, butter, garlic, parsley, salt, and pepper in the crockpot. Stir thoroughly. Put the shrimp in, mixing well. Cook within 1 hour and 30 minutes. Serve.

Nutrition:

- Calories: 250
- Fat: 13.7g
- Carb: 4.6g
- Protein: 27g

6.   Curry Beef

Preparation time: 15 minutes

Cooking time: 8 hours

Servings: 6

Ingredients:

- 1 cup diced tomatoes

- 1 (14-ounce) can coconut milk

- 1/3 cup water

- ¼ cup coconut oil, melted

- ¼ cup tomato paste

- 1 onion, diced

- 6 garlic cloves, minced

- 3 tablespoons grated fresh ginger

- 2 tablespoons ground cumin

- 1 teaspoon paprika

- 1 teaspoon kosher salt

- ½ teaspoon ground turmeric

- ½ teaspoon ground cardamom

- ½ teaspoon ground cinnamon

- ½ teaspoon ground cloves

- ½ teaspoon cayenne pepper

- ¼ teaspoon ground nutmeg

- 1 (1½-pound) beef chuck roast, cut into ½-by-2-inch strips

- 1/3 cup chopped fresh cilantro

Directions:

1. In the slow cooker, stir the tomatoes, coconut milk, water, coconut oil, and tomato paste. Add the onion, garlic, ginger, cumin, paprika, salt, turmeric, cardamom, cinnamon, cloves, cayenne, and nutmeg.

2. Add the beef and toss to mix well. Cover and cook within 8 hours on low. Serve hot, garnished with the cilantro.

Nutrition:

- Calories: 547
- Fat: 46g
- Carbs: 12g
- Protein: 26g

7.   Heavy Creamy Herb Pork Chops

Preparation time: 15 minutes

Cooking time: 8 hours

Servings: 4

Ingredients:

- ¾ cup chicken or beef broth

- 2 tablespoons coconut oil, melted

- 1 tablespoon Dijon mustard

- 2 garlic cloves, minced

- 1 tablespoon paprika

- 1 tablespoon onion powder

- 1 teaspoon dried oregano

- 1 teaspoon dried basil

- 1 teaspoon dried parsley

- 1 onion, thinly sliced

- 4 thick-cut boneless pork chops

- 1 cup heavy (whipping) cream

Directions:

1. In the slow cooker, stir the broth, coconut oil, mustard, garlic, paprika, onion powder, oregano, basil, and parsley.

2.   Add the onion and pork chops and toss to coat. Cover and cook within 8 hours on low or 4 hours on high. Transfer the chops to a serving platter.

3.   Transfer the remaining juices and onion in the slow cooker to a blender, add the heavy cream, and process until smooth. Put the sauce over the pork chops, then serve hot.

Nutrition:

- Calories: 470
- Fat: 32g
- Carbs: 7g
- Protein: 39g

8.   Mushroom Beef Stroganoff

Preparation time: 15 minutes

Cooking time: 8 hours

Servings: 6

Ingredients:

- 2 pounds beef stew meat, cut into 1-inch cubes

- 4 bacon slices, diced

- 8 ounces cremini or button mushrooms, quartered

- 1 onion, halved and sliced

- 2 garlic cloves, minced

- 1 cup beef broth

- ¼ cup tomato paste

- 1 teaspoon smoked paprika

- ½ teaspoon kosher salt

- ¼ teaspoon freshly ground black pepper

- 1½ cups sour cream

- 2 tablespoons minced fresh parsley

Directions:

1. In the slow cooker, stir the beef, bacon, mushrooms, onion, garlic, beef broth, tomato paste, paprika, salt, and pepper. Cover

and cook within 8 hours on low. Stir in the sour cream, then serve hot, garnished with the parsley.

Nutrition:

- Calories: 594
- Fat: 47g
- Carb: 7g
- Protein: 35g

9. Ginger Cream Sauce Pork Loin

Preparation time: 15 minutes

Cooking time: 8 hours

Servings: 6

Ingredients:

For the pork:

- 1 tablespoon erythritol

- 2 teaspoons kosher salt

- 1 teaspoon garlic powder

- 1 teaspoon ground ginger

- ½ teaspoon ground cinnamon

- ½ teaspoon ground cloves

- ½ teaspoon red pepper flakes

- ¼ teaspoon freshly ground black pepper

- 1 (2-pound) pork shoulder roast

- ½ cup of water

For the sauce:

- 2 tablespoons unsalted butter

- 3 tablespoons minced fresh ginger

- 2 shallots, minced

- 1 tablespoon minced garlic

- 2/3 cup dry white wine

- 1 cup heavy (whipping) cream

Directions:

1. In a small bowl, stir the erythritol, salt, garlic powder, ginger, cinnamon, cloves, red pepper flakes, and black pepper. Rub the seasoning mixture all over the pork and place it in the slow cooker.

2. Pour the water into the cooker around the pork. Cover and cook within 8 hours on low. Remove, then let it rest for about 5 minutes.

3. While the pork rests, melt the butter in a small saucepan over medium heat. Stir in the ginger, shallots, and garlic.

4. Add the white wine and bring to a boil. Cook, stirring, until the liquid is reduced to about ¼ cup, about 5 minutes.

5. Mix in the heavy cream, then continue to boil, stirring until the sauce thickens, 3 to 5 minutes more. Slice the pork and serve it with the sauce spooned over the top.

Nutrition:

- Calories: 488
- Fat: 40g
- Carb: 5g
- Protein: 27g

CHAPTER 7:

Mains

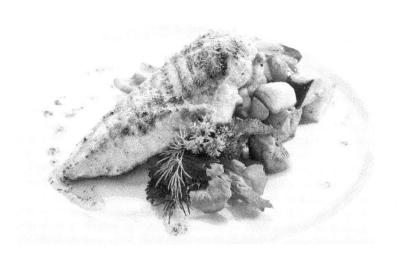

10.   Italian Vegetable Bake

Preparation Time: 15 minutes

Cooking Time: 5 hours

Servings: 7

Ingredients:

- 3 garlic cloves

- 1 can tomato

- 1 bunch oregano

- ¼ tsp. chili flakes

- 11oz. baby aubergines

- 2 Courgettes

- ½ jar roasted red peppers

- 3 tomatoes

- 1 bunch basil

- Green salad

Directions:

1. Peel the garlic and mince. Chop tomatoes from the can. Wash the courgettes and slice, chop baby aubergines. Slice tomatoes. Open the crockpot, put the garlic, diced tomatoes, oregano leaves, chili, and some seasoning, add olive oil if necessary.

2. Add chopped aubergines, tomatoes, courgettes, red peppers, basil, and remaining oregano. Repeat vegetable layer, herb, and

tomatoes. Push down well to compress, set on high for 5 hours. Serve with the basil leaves and the green salad.

Nutrition:

- Calories: 60
- Fat: 3.5g
- Protein: 2g
- Carbs: 6g

11.   Spicy Maple Meatballs

Preparation Time: 15 minutes

Cooking Time: 5 hours

Servings: 11

Ingredients:

- 1 tbsp. olive oil

- ½ white onion

- 1 red bell pepper

- 1 green bell pepper

- 2 jalapeno peppers

- 1½ c. plain tomato sauce

- 1 c. maple syrup

- 2 tbsps. almond flour

- 2 tsp. ground allspice

- 1/8 tsp. liquid smoke

- 1 bag frozen vegan meatballs

Directions:

1. Peel the onion, chop it finely. Wash and slice peppers. Set aside. Add olive oil to the crockpot, add onion and peppers.

2. Take a medium bowl to add flour, maple syrup, tomato sauce, allspice, liquid smoke. Mix all until smooth consistency. Pour into the crockpot.

3. Add frozen meatballs. Cover and cook on low for 5 hours. The sauce should be thick and cover the meatballs. Serve warm over cauliflower rice.

Nutrition:

- Calories: 68
- Fat: 1.6g
- Protein: 7.2g
- Carbs: 6.6g

12.   Vegan Rice and Beans

Preparation Time: 5 minutes

Cooking Time: 4 hours

Servings: 6

Ingredients:

- 2 packages frozen cauliflower rice (12oz each.)
- 2 cans black soybeans, drained
- 1/2 cup hulled hemp seeds
- 1 cup vegetable broth or stock
- 3 tbsp olive oil
- 2 tsp garlic powder
- 1 tsp onion powder
- 1 tsp cumin
- 1 tsp chili powder
- 1/2 tsp cayenne powder
- 1 tbsp Mexican oregano
- Garnishes of choice

Directions:

1. Add all the fixing except the Mexican oregano to the slow cooker, then mix around as best as possible. Let cook on High

within 3-4 hours, until the "rice" is tender. Stir in oregano, then serve.

Nutrition:

- Calories: 299
- Fat: 20.2g
- Protein: 19.3g
- Carbs: 4.9g

CHAPTER 8:

Side Dishes

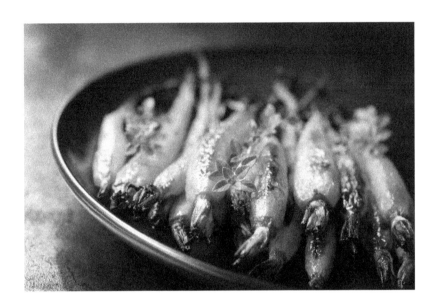

13. Cauliflower Rice

Preparation time: 15 minutes

Cooking time: 2 hours

Servings: 5

Ingredients:

- 1-pound cauliflower

- 1 teaspoon salt

- 1 tablespoon turmeric

- 1 tablespoon butter

- ¾ cup of water

Directions:

1. Chop the cauliflower into tiny pieces to make cauliflower rice. You can also pulse in a food processor to get very fine grains of 'rice'

2. Place the cauliflower rice in the slow cooker. Add salt, turmeric, and water. Stir gently and close the lid. Cook the cauliflower rice for 2 hours on High. Strain the cauliflower rice and transfer it to a bowl. Add butter and stir gently. Serve it!

Nutrition:

- Calories: 48
- Fat: 2.5
- Carbs: 5.7
- Protein: 1.9

14.   Curry Cauliflower

Preparation time: 15 minutes

Cooking time: 5 hours

Servings: 2

Ingredients:

- 10oz. cauliflower

- 1 teaspoon curry paste

- 1 teaspoon curry powder

- ½ teaspoon dried cilantro

- 1oz. butter

- ¾ cup of water

- ¼ cup chicken stock

Directions:

1. Chop the cauliflower roughly and sprinkle it with the curry powder and dried cilantro. Place the chopped cauliflower in the slow cooker. Mix the curry paste with the water. Add chicken stock and transfer the liquid to the slow cooker.

2. Add butter and close the lid. Cook the cauliflower for 5 hours on low. Strain ½ of the liquid off and discard. Transfer the cauliflower to serving bowls. Serve it!

Nutrition:

- Calories: 158 Fat: 13.3g
- Carbs: 8.9g Protein: 3.3g

15. Garlic Cauliflower Steaks

Preparation time: 15 minutes

Cooking time: 3 hours

Servings: 4

Ingredients:

- 14oz. cauliflower head

- 1 teaspoon minced garlic

- 4 tablespoons butter

- 4 tablespoons water

- 1 teaspoon paprika

Directions:

1. Wash the cauliflower head carefully and slice it into the medium steaks. Mix up the butter, minced garlic, and paprika.

2. Rub the cauliflower steaks with the butter mixture. Pour the water into the slow cooker. Add the cauliflower steaks and close the lid.

3. Cook the vegetables for 3 hours on High. Transfer the cooked cauliflower steaks to a platter and serve them immediately!

Nutrition:

- Calories: 129
- Fat: 11.7g
- Carbs: 5.8g
- Protein: 2.2g

16.   Zucchini Gratin

Preparation time: 10 minutes

Cooking time: 5 hours

Servings: 3

Ingredients:

- 1 zucchini, sliced

- 3oz. Parmesan, grated

- 1 teaspoon ground black pepper

- 1 tablespoon butter

- ½ cup almond milk

Directions:

1. Sprinkle the sliced zucchini with the ground black pepper. Chop the butter and place it in the slow cooker.

2. Transfer the sliced zucchini to the slow cooker to make the bottom layer. Add the almond milk. Sprinkle the zucchini with the grated cheese and close the lid.

3. Cook the gratin for 5 hours on low. Then let the gratin cool until room temperature. Serve it!

Nutrition:

- Calories: 229
- Fat: 19.6g
- Carbs: 5.9g
- Protein: 10.9g

CHAPTER 9:

Appetizers

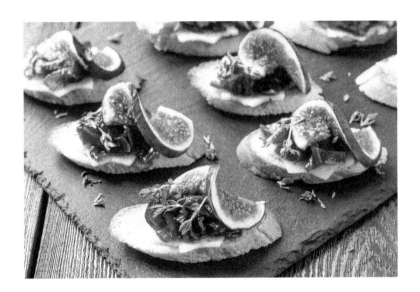

17.   Eggplant and Tomato Salsa

Preparation time: 15 minutes

Cooking time: 7 hours

Servings: 4

Ingredients:

- 1 ½ cup of chopped tomatoes

- 3 cups of cubed eggplant

- 2 tsp. capers

- 6oz. sliced green olives

- 4 minced garlic cloves

- 2 tsp. balsamic vinegar

- 1 tbsp. chopped basil

- Salt

- Black pepper

Directions:

1. In your Slow cooker, mix tomatoes with eggplant, capers, green olives, garlic, vinegar, basil, salt and pepper, toss, cover, and cook on low for 7 hours. Divide salsa into small bowls and serve as an appetizer. Enjoy!

Nutrition:

- Calories: 200 Fat: 6g
- Carbs: 9g Protein: 2g

18.   Carrots and Cauliflower Spread

Preparation time: 15 minutes

Cooking time: 7 hours

Servings: 4

Ingredients:

- 1 cup of sliced carrots

- 1½ cup of cauliflower florets

- 1/3 cup of cashews

- ½ cup of chopped turnips

- 2½ cups of water

- 1 cup of coconut milk

- 1 tsp garlic powder

- ¼ cup of nutritional yeast

- ¼ tsp smoked paprika

- ¼ tsp. mustard powder

- Salt

- Black pepper

Directions:

1. In your slow cooker, mix carrots with cauliflower, cashews, turnips, water, stir, cover, and cook on low for 7 hours.

2. Drain, transfer to a blender, add milk, garlic powder, yeast, paprika, mustard powder, salt, and pepper, blend well, divide into bowls and serve as a party spread. Enjoy!

Nutrition:

- Calories: 291
- Fat: 7g
- Carbs: 14g
- Protein: 3g

19.   Mushroom and Bell Peppers Spread

Preparation time: 15 minutes

Cooking time: 4 hours

Servings: 6

Ingredients:

- 2 c. chopped green bell peppers

- 1 c. chopped yellow onion

- 3 minced garlic cloves

- 1lb. chopped mushrooms

- 28oz. tomato sauce

- Salt

- Black pepper

Directions:

1. In your Slow cooker, mix bell peppers with onion, garlic, mushrooms, tomato sauce, salt and pepper, stir. Cook for 4 hours on low. Divide into bowls and serve as a spread. Enjoy!

Nutrition:

- Calories: 205
- Fat: 4g
- Carbs: 9g
- Protein: 3g

CHAPTER 10:

Seafood

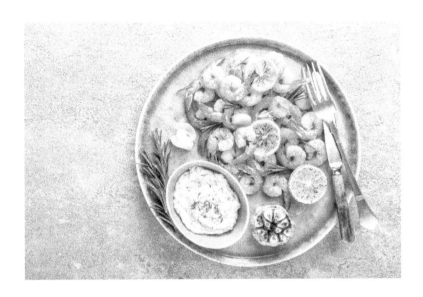

20. Marinara Octopus

Preparation time: 15 minutes

Cooking time: 4 hours

Servings: 4

Ingredients:

- ¼ cup of octopus, cleaned, empty its head

- 2 tablespoons of cherry tomatoes

- 1 clove of garlic, minced

- 1 tablespoon of parsley, minced

- 2 tablespoons of black olives

- 1 pinch of salt

- 1 pinch of black pepper

- 2 tablespoons of olive oil

- 2 tablespoons of capers

For the dip:

- 2 tablespoons of mayonnaise

- 2 tablespoons of sour cream

- 1 tablespoon of ranch seasoning

Directions:

1. Insert in the head of each octopus some minced garlic, parsley (keep some aside), a couple of olives, and 2 capers.

2. At this point, close the heads with a toothpick so that the contents will not come out during cooking. Place half of the cherry tomatoes on the bottom of the Slow Cooker after dicing them

3. Add the olives, the capers, the other part of the chopped parsley, the remaining tomatoes, the tablespoons of oil, salt, and pepper in the bottom of the pot, then place the octopuses on top

4. Close the lid and let it cook within 4 hours by setting the Slow Cooker on high. In the meantime, prepare the dip by combining all of the dip ingredients with a kitchen robot

5. After 4 hours, open the lid. If there is excess liquid, you can cook for another 30/45 minutes with the lid open

Nutrition:

- Calories: 637
- Fat: 57g
- Carbs: 8g
- Protein 31.2g

21. Nagasaki Giant Shrimps

Preparation time: 15 minutes

Cooking time: 4 hours

Servings: 5

Ingredients:

- 5 clean tropical giant shrimps

- 1/3 cup of feta cheese, crumbled

- 1 pinch of onion powder

- 1 pinch of garlic powder

- 1 pinch of pepper

- 2 tablespoons of ripe tomatoes, diced

- 1 tablespoon of tomato paste

- 1 pinch of oregano

- 2 tablespoons olive oil

- 1 pinch of salt

- Parsley or basil leaves to garnish

Directions:

1. Pour the chopped tomatoes, garlic and onion powder, and all seasonings for 5 minutes in a pan with a little oil and then pour it into the Slow Cooker pot.

2. Add tomato sauce, oregano, and salt. Cover and let bake in high mode for 3 hours and a half. In the meanwhile, sauté the shrimps in a pan with a dash of oil.

3. Smear the shrimps with your hands with the ghee to make them soft. Then add the shrimps and let it all cook for another hour with the lid open. In the last half hour, add the crumbled feta and mix it all.

Nutrition:

- Calories: 889
- Fat: 43.15g
- Carbs: 7.6g
- Protein: 27.25g

CHAPTER 11:

Poultry

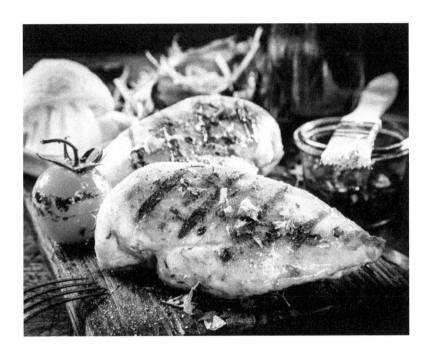

22. Lemongrass and Coconut Chicken Drumsticks

Preparation time: 15 minutes

Cooking Time: 5 hours

Servings: 2

Ingredients:

- 5 chicken drumsticks, skinless

- 1 stalk lemongrass, rough bottom removed

- 1/2 cup coconut milk

- 1/2 tbsp coconut aminos

Directions:

1. Season drumsticks with salt and pepper. Place in the crockpot. In a blender, mix the lemongrass, coconut milk, coconut aminos, garlic and ginger to taste, 1 tbsp fish sauce, and desired spices. Pour the mixture over the drumsticks. Cover and cook on low for 5 hours.

Nutrition:

- Calories: 460
- Fat: 39.7g
- Carbs: 4.7g
- Protein: 36g

23. Bacon & Chicken

Preparation time: 5 minutes

Cooking Time: 8 hours

Servings: 2

Ingredients:

- 1 chicken breasts

- 4 slices of bacon, sliced

- 2 tbsp dried thyme

- 1 tbsp dried oregano

- 1 tbsp dried rosemary

Directions:

1. Mix all ingredients in the crockpot. Add salt to taste. Cook for 8 hours on low. Serve.

Nutrition:

- Calories: 460
- Fat: 39.7g
- Carbs: 4.7g
- Protein: 36g

24.   Roasted Chicken with Lemon & Parsley Butter

Preparation time: 5 minutes

Cooking Time: 8 hours

Servings: 2

Ingredients:

- 4lb. chicken, any part

- 1 whole lemon, sliced

- 2 tbsp butter or ghee

- 1 tbsp parsley, chopped

Directions:

1. Massage chicken all over with salt plus pepper to taste. Put it in the crockpot and pour 1 cup of water. Cover and cook for 3 hours on high.

2. When cooked, add the lemon slices, butter, and parsley to the crockpot. Cook and cover for another 10 minutes.

Nutrition:

- Calories: 300
- Fat: 18g
- Carbs: 1g
- Protein: 29g

25.   Onion and Mushroom Chicken Breasts

Preparation time: 5 minutes

Cooking Time: 8 hours

Servings: 2

Ingredients:

- 1 sliced onion

- 1 cup sliced mushrooms

- 2 chicken breasts

- 1 cup chicken broth

- Thyme

Directions:

1. Place half the onion slices on the bottom of the crockpot and add the chicken on top. Top again with the remainder of onion slices.

2. Add all other ingredients carefully into the crockpot. Add salt and pepper to taste. Cook on low for 8 hours.

Nutrition:

- Calories: 345
- Fat: 29g
- Carbs: 4g
- Protein: 32g

CHAPTER 12:

Meats

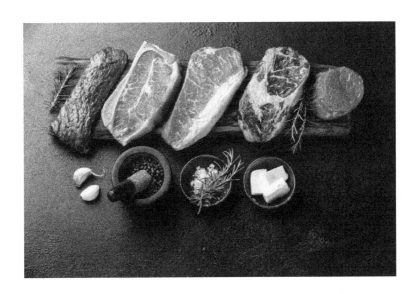

26. North American Pork Ribs

Preparation Time: 20 minutes

Cooking Time: 10 hours

Servings: 6

Ingredients:

- 3 pounds pork ribs

- 1 small yellow onion, chopped

- 2 garlic cloves, minced

- 1 cup baby carrots, peeled and chopped

- ½ cup homemade chicken broth

- ¼ cup coconut aminos

- 1 tablespoon olive oil

- Salt

- Ground black pepper

Directions:

1. In a large crockpot, add all ingredients and stir to combine. Set the crockpot on low and cook, covered, within 8-10 hours. Serve hot.

Nutrition:

- Calories: 506 Carbohydrates: 5.8g
- Protein: 45.9g
- Fat: 32g

27.   Simply Delicious Pork Chops

Preparation Time: 15 minutes **Cooking Time:** 5 hours 5 minutes

Servings: 5

Ingredients:

- 1 tablespoon coconut oil

- 2 garlic cloves, minced

- 5 (4-ounce) boneless pork chops

- Salt

- Ground black pepper

- 1 large zucchini, cubed

- 2 lemons, sliced

- 1 teaspoon red pepper flakes, crushed

Directions:

1. In a large skillet, heat-up oil on medium-high heat and sauté garlic for about 1 minute. Add chops and cook for 1-2 minutes per side.

2. Transfer the chops mixture into a crockpot. Place cubed zucchini over chops evenly, followed by lemon slices.

3. Sprinkle with red pepper flakes, salt, and black pepper. Set the crockpot on High and cook, covered, for about 5 hours. Serve hot

Nutrition:

- Calories: 206 Carbohydrates: 4.9g Protein: 30.8g Fat: 7g

28.   Fall-of-the-Bone Pork Shoulder

Preparation Time: 15 minutes

Cooking Time: 8 hours 10 minutes

Servings: 8

Ingredients:

- 2 tablespoons olive oil
- 3 pounds of pork shoulder
- Salt
- Ground black pepper
- 1 medium yellow onion, chopped
- 1 celery stalk, chopped
- 2 garlic cloves, minced
- 2 cups fresh tomatoes, chopped finely
- ½ cup homemade chicken broth
- 2 tablespoons fresh lemon juice

Directions:

1. In a large skillet, heat-up oil on medium-high heat and cook pork shoulder with salt and black pepper for about 4-5 minutes per side.

2. Transfer pork shoulder to a crockpot and top with onion, celery, garlic, and tomatoes. Pour broth and lemon juice on top.

29.   Christmas Dinner Pork Roast

Preparation Time: 15 minutes **Cooking Time:** 8 hours

Servings: 10

Ingredients:

- 4 pounds boneless pork roast

- 1 teaspoon dried rosemary, crushed

- 1 teaspoon dried thyme, crushed

- 1 teaspoon cayenne pepper

- ½ teaspoon smoked paprika

- Salt

- Ground black pepper

- 1 medium yellow onion, sliced thinly and divided

- 1 cup hot homemade chicken broth

Directions:

1. Rub the pork with herbs and spices generously. At the bottom of a large crockpot, place half the onion and top with pork roast, followed by the remaining onion.

2. Pour broth on top. Set the crockpot on low and cook, covered, for about 6-8 hours. Uncover the crockpot and transfer the pork roast onto a cutting board. Cut pork roast into desired sized slices and serve.

Nutrition:

- Calories: 269 Carbohydrates: 1.4g Protein: 48.1g Fat: 17.5g

3. Set the crockpot on low and cook, covered, for about 8 hours. Uncover the crockpot and transfer the pork shoulder onto a cutting board. Cut pork shoulder into desired sized slices and serve.

Nutrition:

- Calories: 545
- Carbohydrates: 3.5g
- Protein: 40.5g
- Fat: 40.1g

30.   Asian Style Pork Butt

Preparation Time: 15 minutes

Cooking Time: 8 hours

Servings: 8

Ingredients:

- 1 medium onion, sliced thinly

- 4 garlic cloves, minced

- 3 tablespoons lemongrass, minced

- 1 tablespoon vinegar

- 3 tablespoons olive oil

- Salt

- Ground black pepper

- 3 pounds pork butt, trimmed

- 1 cup unsweetened coconut milk

Directions:

1. In a large bowl, add garlic, lemongrass, vinegar, oil, and seasoning. Rub the pork butt with garlic mixture evenly.

2. In a large crockpot, place the onion slices and top with pork butt. Cover the crockpot and set aside to marinate for at least 8 hours.

3. Uncover the crockpot and pour coconut milk on top. Set the crockpot on low and cook, covered, for about 8 hours.

4. Uncover the crockpot and transfer the pork butt onto a cutting board. Cut pork butt into desired sized slices and serve.

Nutrition:

- Calories: 445
- Carbohydrates: 3.9g
- Protein: 53.9g
- Fat: 23.8g

31. Balsamic Dijon Short Ribs

Preparation time: 15 minutes

Cooking time: 8 hours

Servings: 6

Ingredients:

- 2 pounds beef short ribs

- 1 teaspoon salt

- 1 teaspoon black pepper

- 2 tablespoons olive oil

- 2 cups Napa cabbage, shredded

- ¼ cup balsamic vinegar

- ¼ cup Dijon mustard

- ½ cup beef stock

- 1 tablespoon fresh thyme

- 2 garlic cloves, crushed and minced

Directions:

1. Flavor the ribs with salt plus black pepper. Heat-up olive oil in a skillet over medium heat. Place the ribs in the skillet and cook for 1-2 minutes per side.

2. Spread the cabbage in the bottom of the slow cooker. Transfer the ribs from the skillet to the slow cooker.

3. Combine the balsamic vinegar, Dijon mustard, beef stock, thyme, garlic, and mix well. Pour the mixture over the ribs. Cover and cook on low within 8 hours.

Nutrition:

- Calories: 282.1
- Fat: 15.4g
- Carbs: 1.8g
- Protein: 30.4g

CHAPTER 13:

Vegetables

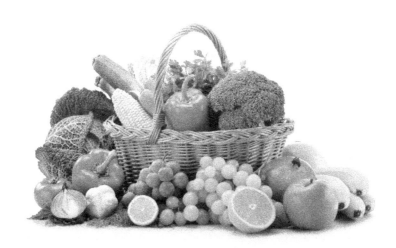

32.   Garlic Herb Mushrooms

Preparation time: 15 minutes

Cooking time: 4 hours

Servings: 4

Ingredients:

- ¼ teaspoon thyme

- 2 bay leaves

- 1 cup vegetable broth

- ½ cup half and half

- 2 tablespoons butter

- 2 tablespoons fresh parsley, chopped

- Salt and pepper, to taste

Directions:

1. Place all of the ingredients save for the butter and the half and half in the slow cooker and put on low for 3 hours. Once done, add the butter and half for the last 15 minutes. Garnish with parsley and enjoy.

Nutrition:

- Calories: 175
- Fat: 18g
- Protein: 3g
- Carbs: 18g

33.   Sticky Sesame Cauliflower Slow Cooker Bites

Preparation time: 15 minutes

Cooking time: 2 hours

Servings: 4

Ingredients:

- 1-pound cauliflower

- ½ teaspoon paprika

- ½ teaspoon ground cumin

- 1 teaspoon garlic powder

- 1 teaspoon sesame oil

- 1/3 cup honey

- 2 tablespoons apple cider vinegar

- 1 teaspoon sweet chili sauce

- 3 garlic cloves, minced

- ¼ cup of water

- 1 tablespoon arrowroot powder or cornstarch

- 1 cup green onions to garnish

- Sesame seeds to garnish

Directions:

1. Place all spices, minus the green onions and sesame seeds, in a bowl, and cover the cauliflower thoroughly with the mixture. Place the cauliflower into the slow cooker.

2. Add the rest of the ingredients and cover. Cook on low for 2 hours. The sauce will thicken with the cornstarch or arrowroot powder. When done, remove each bite and garnish with toasted sesame seeds and green onion slices on top.

Nutrition:

- Calories: 240
- Fat: 7g
- Protein: 3g
- Carbs: 18g

34. Crockpot Cauliflower Mac and Cheese

Preparation time: 15 minutes

Cooking time: 4 hours

Servings: 4

Ingredients:

- 1-pound cauliflower

- 2 cups shredded cheddar cheese

- 2 ½ cups milk

- 1 12-ounce can evaporate milk

- ½ tablespoon mustard

Directions:

1. Place all of the fixings above in the slow cooker and put on low for 3 hours until most of the liquid has been absorbed.

2. Sprinkle some extra cheese on top and cook for 15 minutes until it has melted and the rest of the liquid is absorbed. Garnish with some parsley and even shredded parmesan cheese.

Nutrition:

- Calories: 215
- Fat: 4g
- Protein: 3g
- Carbs: 18g

35.   Crockpot Vegetable Lasagna

Preparation time: 15 minutes

Cooking time: 2 hours

Servings: 4

Ingredients:

- 2 medium zucchinis

- 1 medium eggplant

- 2 cups tomato-based pasta sauce

- 1 red onion, diced

- 1 red bell pepper, diced

- 16 ounces low fat cottage cheese

- 2 large eggs

- 8 ounces shredded Mozzarella

- 2 tablespoons basil, chopped

- 2 tablespoons parmesan cheese, for garnish

Directions:

1. Slice eggplant plus zucchini lengthwise into thin strips, approximately ¼ inch thick so that they resemble the shape of lasagna noodles. Spread them out over a layer of paper towels and toss with salt.

2. Let stand for 15 minutes to absorb the salt. It helps the vegetables to absorb the liquid. Lightly coat the bottom of your crockpot and spread ½ cup of tomato sauce along the bottom.

3. In a separate bowl, beat the eggs and cottage cheese. Create a layer of "noodles," then 1/3 of the cottage cheese mixture, 1/3 of the bell peppers and onions, and 1/3 of the mozzarella and tomato sauce.

4. Put down another layer of "noodles," then repeat. Finish with the third layer of "noodles." Cook on high for 2 hours, until the eggplant is tender. Slice and scoop out portions as desired, then garnish with herbs and cheese.

Nutrition:

- Calories: 213
- Fat: 9g
- Protein: 3g
- Carbs: 18g

36.   Tasty Tagine Five a Day

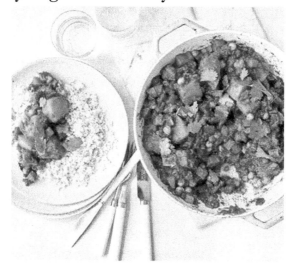

Preparation time: 15 minutes

Cooking time: 8 hours

Servings: 6

Ingredients:

- 4 tablespoons of olive oil

- 1 sliced red onion

- 2 cloves of crushed garlic

- 500 grams of aubergine in 1 cm-thick slice, cut lengthways

- 300 grams of quartered ripe tomatoes

- 1 small sliced fennel bulb

- 50 grams of sundried tomatoes

- 1 teaspoon of coriander seeds

For the dressing:

- 100 grams of feta cheese, and extra for topping

- 50 grams of toasted almond flakes

Directions:

1. Put two tbsp of olive oil into the slow cooker and add the crushed garlic and the onions. Brush the aubergines with the remaining olive oil and place them on top of the onions and garlic.

2. Arrange the sundried tomatoes, fennel slices, and the tomatoes around the aubergines. Flavor it with salt plus pepper and pour the coriander seeds over the top. Cook for 6-8 hours on low.

3. Place the dressing ingredients into a food processor and work until smooth. Spoon the vegetables onto serving dishes, drizzle the dressing over the top and crumble the feta cheese on top.

Nutrition:

- Calories: 289
- Fat: 20g
- Carbs: 11g
- Protein: 8g

CHAPTER 14:

Soups & Stews

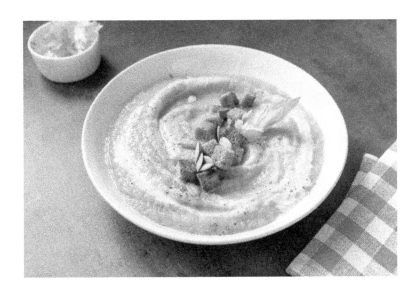

37.   Chicken & Bacon Chowder

Preparation time: 15 minutes

Cooking time: 8 hours

Servings: 8

Ingredients:

- 1 trimmed – sliced leek

- 6oz. sliced cremini mushrooms

- 1 finely chopped shallot

- 1 med. thinly sliced sweet onion

- 4 minced garlic cloves

- 4 tbsp. butter – divided

- 2 diced celery ribs

- 2 cups of chicken stock – divided

- 1 lb. chicken breasts

- 1 pkg. (8oz.) cream cheese

- 1 lb. bacon – crispy & crumbled

- 1 cup of heavy cream

1 tsp of each:

- Sea salt

- Dried thyme

- Black pepper

- Garlic powder

Directions:

1. Using the low setting for one hour, add the shallot, garlic, leek, mushrooms, celery, onions, one cup of the chicken stock, black pepper, sea salt, and two tablespoons butter to the slow cooker. Secure the lid.

2. In a skillet, sear the chicken breasts over the med-high setting on the stovetop using the rest of the butter. It should take approximately five minutes per side—making sure they are browned evenly. Set aside on a platter.

3. Deglaze the pan with the rest of the stock using a rubber spatula. Add the chicken to the slow cooker and pour in the cream, garlic powder, thyme, and cream cheese. Combine the mixture until the chunks of cheese are consumed in the mixture.

4. After the chicken has cooled down, cut it into cubes, and toss it into the cooker along with the bacon. Mix well. Cover and simmer for six to eight hours (low). When done, serve, and enjoy.

Nutrition:

- Calories: 355
- Carbs: 5.75g
- Fat: 28g
- Protein: 21g

38.   Kale & Chicken Soup

Preparation time: 15 minutes

Cooking time: 6 hours

Servings: 6

Ingredients:

- 2lb. chicken thighs/breast meat

- 1/3 cup of onion

- ½ cup (+) 1 tbsp. olive oil

- 14oz. chicken broth

- 32oz. chicken stock

- 5oz. baby kale leaves

- Salt & pepper to taste

- ¼ cup of lemon juice

Also Needed:

- Large skillet

- Blender

Directions:

1.   Remove all skin, including bones, from the chicken. Dice the onions. Heat-up one tbsp of the oil in a frying pan (med. heat). Sprinkle the pepper and salt on the chicken. Toss it into the pan.

2. Lower the temperature to med-low and cover. Continue cooking the chicken until it reaches the internal temperature of 165°F (approximately 15 minutes).

3. Shred your cooked chicken, and add it to the slow cooker. Use the blender to combine the rest of the oil, onion, and chicken broth.

4. Scrape it into the cooker. Stir in the rest of the ingredients and cover. Prepare for 6 hours. Stir a few times during the final cycle. Serve and enjoy.

Nutrition:

- Calories: 261
- Carbs: 2g
- Protein: 14.1g
- Fat: 21g

39.   Reuben Soup with Thousand Island Dressing

Preparation time: 15 minutes

Cooking time: 8 hours

Servings: 12

Ingredients:

- 1 medium diced onion

- 8 cups of beef broth/stock

- 3 minced garlic cloves

- 2 tbsp. butter

- 2lbs. diced corned beef

- 1 lb. Sauerkraut

- 1 tbsp. mustard seeds

1 tsp of each:

- Dill seeds

- Coriander seeds

1 Hour Before Serving:

- 8oz. shredded Swiss cheese

- 2 cups of heavy cream

For the Topping:

- Thousand Island dressing

Directions:

1. Use the medium heat setting to brown the onion and garlic using one tablespoon of butter. Sauté for two minutes.

2. Stir in the beef broth, remaining butter, garlic, onions, mustard seeds, sauerkraut, corned beef, and beef broth. Prepare the soup using the high setting for 3.5 hours or 7 hours on low.

3. Approximately one hour before dinner, add the whipping cream and Swiss cheese. Top if off with the Thousand Island dressing as desired.

Nutrition:

- Calories: 343
- Carb: 1.3g
- Fat: 25.6g
- Protein: 22.8g

40. Sausage & Pepper Soup

Preparation time: 15 minutes

Cooking time: 5 hours

Servings: 4

Ingredients:

- 1 ½ lb. hot Italian sausage

- 2 cups of beef stock

- 6 cups of raw spinach

- ½ med. onion

- 1 medium of each: red & green bell pepper

- 1 can tomato with jalapenos

- ½ tsp kosher salt

2 tsp of each:

- Minced garlic

- Cumin

- Chili powder

- 1 tsp Italian seasoning

Directions:

1. Break the sausage into chunks and cook. Slice the green peppers. Toss the peppers, stock, and spices into the slow cooker. Arrange the sausage on top and mix well.

2. Fry the garlic and onions and add to the slow cooker. Toss the spinach and prepare using the high setting for three hours. Stir, and reduce the heat to the low setting for another two hours of cooking. Stir and serve.

Nutrition:

- Calories: 612.25
- Protein: 27.11g
- Carbs: 7.81g
- Fat: 50.79g

41.   Spring Keto Stew with Venison

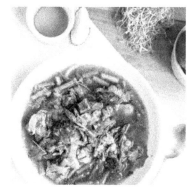

Preparation time: 20 minutes

Cooking Time: 6 hours

Servings: 2

Ingredients:

- 1lb. venison stew meat

- 1/2 cup purple cabbage, shredded

- 1/2 cup celery, sliced

- 2 cup bone broth

Directions:

1. Sauté cabbage and celery with olive oil and garlic in a skillet. Add the venison and season with salt and pepper to taste. Stir until meat is browned. Transfer everything into the crockpot. Add the cone broth. Cover and cook on low for 6 hours.

Nutrition:

- Calories: 310 Fat: 16g
- Carbs: 5g Protein: 32g

CHAPTER 15:

Condiments

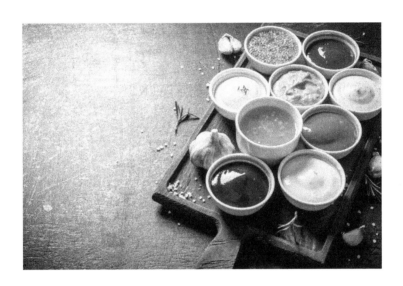

42. Easy BBQ Sauce

Preparation time: 15 minutes

Cooking time: 8 hours

Servings: 4

Ingredients:

- 8-ounces canned no-sugar tomato sauce
- 2 tablespoons no-sugar Worcestershire sauce
- 2 tablespoons apple cider vinegar
- 2 tablespoons stone-ground mustard
- 1 tablespoon onion powder
- 1 tablespoon chili powder
- 2 teaspoons liquid smoke
- ¼ teaspoon garlic powder
- ½ teaspoon liquid stevia
- 1 teaspoon of sea salt
- Dash of black pepper

Directions:

1. Put all the listed fixing in your slow cooker. Cook on low within 6-8 hours. When time is up, use right away!

Nutrition:

- Calories: 56 Protein: 1g Carbs: 11g Fat: 0g

43.   Asian-Inspired BBQ Sauce

Preparation time: 15 minutes

Cooking time: 8 hours

Servings: 1

Ingredients:

- ¾ cup coconut aminos

- 6 tablespoons no-sugar tomato paste

- 6 tablespoons melted unsweetened almond butter

- 3 tablespoons apple cider vinegar

- 4 minced garlic cloves

- 3 teaspoons Dijon mustard

- 1 ½ teaspoons paprika

- Generous pinch of cinnamon

- Salt and pepper to taste

Directions:

1. Put all the fixing in your slow cooker. Cook on low for 6-8 hours. Use!

Nutrition:

- Calories: 105
- Protein: 3g
- Carbs: 9g
- Fat: 7g

CHAPTER 16:

Snacks

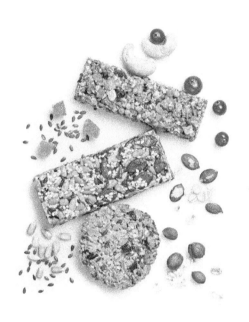

44.   Cauliflower Hummus

Preparation time: 15 minutes

Cooking time: 4 hours

Servings: 8

Ingredients:

- 3 cups cauliflower florets

- 5 garlic cloves, peeled

- 1 1/2 tablespoons tahini paste

- 2 tablespoons olive oil

- 3 tablespoons lemon juice

Directions:

1. Place the cauliflower florets in a 4-quart slow-cooker, add 3 garlic cloves and 1/4 cup water, and season with a pinch of salt.

2. Cover and seal the slow-cooker with its lid, and adjust the cooking timer for 3 to 4 hours. Allow cooking at a low heat setting.

3. Pulse the cauliflower mixture with a stick blender until smooth. Add the remaining ingredients and pulse again with a stick blender until smooth. Adjust the seasoning, drizzle with olive oil and serve with chopped vegetables.

Nutrition:

- Calories: 141 Carbohydrates: 7g
- Fats: 14g
- Protein: 2g

45.   'Powerful 4' Chicken Wings

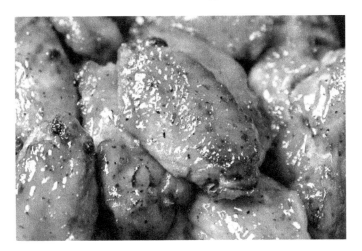

Preparation time: 15 minutes

Cooking time: 4 hours

Servings: 6

Ingredients:

- 6 chicken fillets

- 1 bottle hot sauce

- 4 tbsp butter, melted

- ½ packet ranch seasoning

Directions:

1.   Make a mixture of hot sauce plus ranch seasoning, then coat the chicken pieces with it. Dissolve the butter in the slow-cooker, then put the chicken pieces at the bottom.

2. Cook without the lid for the first 30 minutes and then cook with the cover on a low setting for 3 hours 30 minutes. Serve with some of your favorite vegetables and sauce.

Nutrition:

- Calories: 140
- Carbs: 0g
- Fat: 18g
- Protein: 21g

46.   Lamb Fillet

Preparation time: 15 minutes

Cooking time: 5 hours

Servings: 6

Ingredients:

- 6 lamb fillets, cut into ½ inch thick pieces

- 1 bottle hot sauce

- ½ cup tomato ketchup

- 4 tbsp butter, melted

- ½ packet ranch seasoning

Directions:

1. Make a mixture of hot sauce plus ranch seasoning and thoroughly coat the chicken pieces with it. Dissolve the butter in the slow cooker and place the chicken pieces at the bottom.

2. Cook without the lid within 30 minutes and then cook with the cover on low within 4 hours 30 minutes. Serve with some of your favorite vegetables and sauce.

Nutrition:

- Calories: 135
- Carbs: 0g
- Fat: 7g
- Protein: 27g

47. Chicken Rolls with Bean Sprouts

Preparation time: 15 minutes **Cooking time:** 4 hours

Servings: 4

Ingredients:

- 4lb. chicken breast fillets

- 1 bunch asparagus, finely chopped

- 2 cloves of minced garlic

- 1 cup green beans sprout

- 1 cup grated mozzarella cheese

- 1 tsp salt

- 3 tbsp olive oil

- 1 tsp pepper

Directions:

1. Flatten the chicken fillets on the table using a wooden hammer. Put the green bean sprouts, garlic, salt, pepper, asparagus, plus grated cheese in a bowl and blend them properly.

2. Split the batter equally in 4 chicken fillets and cover the chicken tightly and secure with wooden toothpicks.

3. Put the chicken rolls in the slow cooker and cook on the low setting within 4 hours. Serve hot with your favorite sauce.

Nutrition:

- Calories: 150 Carbs: 14g
- Fat: 7g Protein: 8g

CHAPTER 17:

Desserts

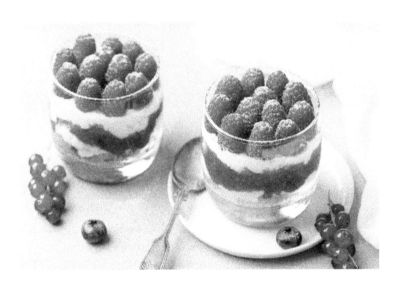

48.   Keto Cheesecake

Preparation time: 15 minutes

Cooking time: 3 hours

Servings: 12

Ingredients:

- ½ tbsp. vanilla extract

- 1 cup of Splenda

- 3 8-ounce packages of cream cheese

- 3 eggs

Directions:

1. Let the cream cheese to warm up at room temperature. Mix sugar and cream cheese until well blended. Mix in one egg at a time, making sure to beat well after every addition.

2. Add vanilla and mix well. Grease a pan or bowl well and add cream cheese mixture to it. Add 2-3 cups of water into the bottom of the slow cooker. Add pan to pot. Set to cook on high 2 – 2 ½ hours.

Nutrition:

- Calories: 301
- Carbs: 2g
- Fat: 31g
- Protein: 23g

49.   Creamy Pumpkin Custard

Preparation time: 15 minutes **Cooking time:** 3 hours

Servings: 10

Ingredients:

- 4 tbsp. butter

- 1 tsp. pumpkin pie spice

- ½ cup of almond flour

- 1 tsp. vanilla extract

- 1 cup of pumpkin puree

- ½ cup of granulated stevia

- 4 eggs

- 1/8 tsp. salt

Directions:

1. Grease inside of a slow cooker. Beat eggs until smooth. Then beat in sweetener gradually. Add vanilla and pumpkin puree until blended well.

2. Then mix in pumpkin pie spice, salt, and almond flour. Blend as you add in butter. Pour into a slow cooker.

3. Place a paper towel over the opening of the pot before closing it. Cook 2-3 hours on low. Serve warm with whipped cream and a dash of nutmeg!

Nutrition:

- Calories: 419 Carbs: 4g Fat: 16g Protein: 19g

50. Chocolate Molten Lava Cake

Preparation time: 15 minutes

Cooking time: 3 hours

Servings: 12

Ingredients:

- ½ cup of melted and cooled butter

- ½ cup of flour

- ½ tsp. salt

- ½ tsp. vanilla liquid stevia

- 1 ½ cup of swerve sweetener

- 1 tsp. baking powder

- 1 tsp. vanilla extract

- 2 cups of hot water

- 3 egg yolks

- 3 whole eggs

- 4-ounces sugar-free chocolate chips

- 5 tbsp. unsweetened cocoa powder

Directions:

1. Grease slow cooker liberally. Whisk baking powder, salt, 3 tbsp cocoa powder, flour, and 1 ¼ cup of swerve sweetener. Stir liquid stevia, vanilla, yolks, eggs, and melted butter.

2. Combine wet and dry mixture till well incorporated. Pour into a slow cooker. Top with chocolate chips. Mix in the remaining swerve and cocoa powder. Set to cook on low 3 hours.

Nutrition:

- Calories: 418
- Carbs: 4g
- Fat: 27g
- Protein: 8g

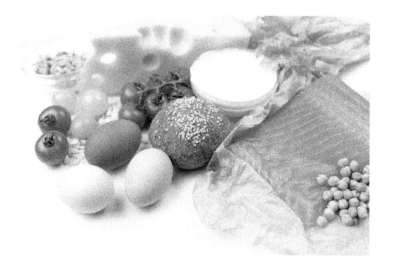

Conclusion

N ow you can cook healthier meals for yourself, your family, and your friends to get your metabolism running at the peak of perfection and help you feel healthy, lose weight, and maintain a healthy balanced diet. And it all thanks to the combination of the Keto diet and your amazing slow cooker in this cookbook! A new diet isn't so bad when you have so many options from which to choose. You may miss your carbs, but with all these tasty recipes at your fingertips, you'll find them easily replaced with new favorites.

You will marvel at how much energy you have after sweating through the first week or so of almost no carbs. It can be a challenge, but you can do it! Pretty soon, you won't miss those things that bogged down your metabolism as well as your thinking and made you tired and cranky. You will feel like you can rule the world and do anything once your body is purged of heavy carbs, and you start eating things that rejuvenate your body. It is worth a few detox symptoms when you start enjoying the food you are eating.

A keto diet isn't one that you can keep going on and off. It will take your body a little some time to get adjusted and for ketosis to set in. This process could take anywhere between two to seven days. It depends on the level of activity, body type, and the food you are eating.

There are various mobile applications that you can make use of for tracking your carbohydrate intake. There are paid and free applications as well. These apps will help you in keeping track of your total carbohydrate and fiber intake. However, you won't be able to track your net carb intake. MyFitnessPal is one of the popular apps. You need to open the app store on your smartphone, and you can select an app from the various available apps.

The weight that you will lose will depend on you. If you add exercise to your daily routine, then the weight loss will be more significant. If you cut down on foods that stall weight loss, then this will speed up the process. For instance, completely cutting out things like artificial sweeteners, dairy, wheat products, and other related products will help speed up your weight loss. During your first two weeks of the keto diet, you will end up losing all the excess water weight. Ketosis has a diuretic effect on the body, and you might end up losing a couple of pounds within the first few days of this diet. After this, your body will adapt itself to burning fats to generate energy instead of carbs.

You now have everything you need to break free from a dependence on highly processed foods, with all their dangerous additives that your body interprets as toxins. You can still enjoy your favorite pasta dishes, even taco salad, but without the grogginess in the afternoon that comes with all those unnecessary carbs.

So, energize your life and sustain a healthy body by applying what you've discovered. You don't have to change everything at once. Just start by adopting a new recipe each week that sounds interesting to you.

Gradually, swap out less-than-healthy options for ingredients and recipes from this book that will promote your well-being. Each time you make a healthy substitution or try a new ketogenic recipe, you can feel proud of yourself; you are taking good care of your mind and body. Even before you start to experience the benefits of a ketogenic lifestyle, you can feel good because you are choosing the best course for your life.

Thanks for reading!

CPSIA information can be obtained
at www.ICGtesting.com
Printed in the USA
BVHW041628230221
600894BV00014B/1318

9 781801 764902